CKD SOLUTION DIET COOKBOOK
FOR ALL STAGES

Are you ready for A New Life, A new special
365day recipes for ckd treatment, Plus
30day meal plan to stay fitness today.

Dr. D. SAM

TABLE OF CONTENT

INTRODUCTION

Introducing our CKD Diet Cookbook for All Stages: Your Comprehensive Guide to Delicious and Kidney-Friendly Meals!

Navigating the dietary restrictions of chronic kidney disease (CKD) can be overwhelming, but with our cookbook, managing your condition has never been easier or more enjoyable.

Designed to cater to individuals across all stages of CKD, our cookbook offers a diverse collection of recipes carefully crafted to support kidney health while tantalizing your taste buds. From hearty breakfast options to satisfying dinners, and even snacks and desserts, each recipe is thoughtfully curated to prioritize nutrient balance and flavor without compromising on dietary restrictions.

Whether you're newly diagnosed or a seasoned CKD warrior, our cookbook provides the tools and inspiration you need to take control of your diet and optimize your well-being. Say goodbye to bland meals and hello to a world of culinary delight with our CKD Diet Cookbook for All Stages!

WHAT IS RENAL ILLNESS THAT IS CHRONIC?

A chronic illness known as chronic kidney disease (CKD) is characterized by a progressive loss of kidney function over time. The kidneys are essential organs that filter waste materials and extra fluid from the blood, excreting them in the urine. Waste materials and fluids can accumulate in the body as a result of declining kidney function, which can cause a number of health issues.

Stages of Chronic Kidney Disease (CKD) The glomerular filtration rate (GFR), a measure of how well the kidneys filter blood, divides CKD into five stages:

Stage 1: Kidney injury with a GFR of 90 mL/min or greater and either normal or high

Stage 2: Mildly decreased GFR (60-89 mL/min) due to kidney injury

Stahe 3: Moderately decreased GFR (30–59 mL/min) is stage three.

Stage 4: GFR significantly decreased (15–29 mL/min)

Stage 5: End-stage renal disease (ESRD) or kidney failure (GFR < 15 mL/min), necessitating kidney transplantation or dialysis.

Reasons

A number of illnesses can result in CKD, such as:

Diabetes: Over time, kidney damage can result from high blood sugar levels.

Hypertension: Elevated blood pressure has the potential to harm kidney blood vessels.

Inflammation of the kidney's glomeruli, or filtering units, is known as glomerulonephritis.

Kidney cyst formation is a hereditary illness known as polycystic kidney disease.

Long-term obstruction: Blockages in the urinary system caused by tumors, enlarged prostates, or kidney stones.

Recurrent kidney infections: Kidney damage can result from long-term pyelonephritis.

Signs and symptoms

Symptoms are frequently absent in the early stages of CKD. As the illness worsens, possible symptoms include:

Weakness and exhaustion

Edema, or swelling in the legs, ankles, or feet

Breathlessness

vomiting and nausea

appetite decline
alterations in the look and production of urine
twitches and spasms of muscles
Continuous itching
Diagnosis: CKD is identified by:

Blood tests: To calculate GFR and quantify creatinine.
Tests on pee: To look for blood or protein in the urine.
Imaging tests: CT or ultrasound scans to see the anatomy of the kidneys.
Kidney biopsy: A tiny sample of kidney tissue may be removed for analysis in certain circumstances.
Handling and Medical Interventions
Although there isn't a cure for CKD, therapy aims to alleviate symptoms and limit the disease's progression:

Medication: To regulate cholesterol, blood sugar, and blood pressure.

Dietary adjustments: Cutting back on potassium, protein, and salt.

Dialysis: An advanced stage treatment that takes over the kidneys' functions when they fail.

Kidney transplant: Using a healthy kidney from a donor to replace a damaged kidney.

Avoidance

Managing risk factors is necessary to prevent CKD:

Manage diabetes and high blood pressure: using medicine, food, and way of life adjustments.

Keep your weight in check with a balanced diet and frequent exercise.

Refrain from drinking too much alcohol and smoking.

Frequent check-ups: For people who are at risk, like those who have high blood pressure or diabetes.

For the purpose of controlling CKD and enhancing quality of life, early detection and treatment are essential.

Depending on the stage of the condition, different foods are advised for people with chronic kidney disease (CKD). The broad guidelines for foods to limit or avoid at each stage are listed below:

All-Ages General Dietary Guidelines
Limiting sodium consumption can help lower blood pressure and lessen fluid retention. Steer clear of restaurant meals, processed foods, canned soups, and salty snacks.
Phosphorus: Excessive phosphorus intake can cause heart and bone issues. Limit your intake of bran cereals, colas, beans, lentils, nuts, seeds, and dairy products.

Potassium: Elevated potassium levels may have an impact on heart health. Eat less spinach, oranges, potatoes, bananas, and tomatoes.

Protein: To lessen the strain on the kidneys as CKD worsens, protein consumption may need to be restricted. Select healthy proteins in moderation, such as lean meat, fish, eggs, and dairy.

Stages 1 and 2 of CKD

During the initial phases, the emphasis is on upholding a nutritious diet and managing blood pressure and glucose levels. Generally, there is no need for substantial dietary restrictions; the key is moderation.

Moderate consumption of protein.

Don't take more than 2,300 mg of sodium daily.

Potassium and phosphorus: Usually not restricted, but may need to be monitored.

Stage 3 CKD

More targeted dietary changes are required when renal function deteriorates:

Protein: Keep daily consumption to 0.8 grams per kilogram of body weight.

Limit your daily sodium intake to 1,500–2,300 mg.

Start limiting foods that are high in phosphorus.

Potassium: Adjust your consumption to your blood level.

Stage 4 CKD

More severe dietary restrictions are implemented to control symptoms and decrease the progression of the disease:

Additional restriction on protein intake: 0.6-0.75 grams per kilogram of body weight each day.

Keep your daily sodium intake at 1,500–2,300 mg.

Phosphorus: Limit consumption even more.

Potassium: Keep an eye on it and set limits according to blood levels.

Fluids: If you're swollen or having trouble breathing, you might need to cut back on your fluid consumption.

Stage 5 CKD (End-Stage Renal Disease): Dietary restrictions are stringent, and patients frequently need dialysis:

Consumption of protein is contingent upon the patient's dialysis status. Patients on dialysis might require more protein.

Limit sodium intake strictly to no more than 2,000 mg daily.

Phosphorus: Steer clear of foods high in phosphorus and, if directed, take phosphate binders.

Potassium: strictly restrict consumption and keep a close eye on blood levels.

Fluids: Limit according to dialysis schedule and urine production.

Foods to Refrain from or Reduce

Foods High in Sodium

processed meats, such as deli, sausage, and bacon

canned veggies and soups

salty appetizers (pretzels, chips)
Fast food and dinners from restaurants
Olives and pickles
Other condiments high in sodium, such as soy sauce
Foods High in Phosphorus
dairy goods, such as cheese, yogurt, and milk
Seeds and nuts
Lentils with beans
oatmeal and bran cereals
Dark-colored drinks and colas
Foods High in Potassium
Orange juice, bananas, and oranges
Sweet potatoes with potatoes
Tomatoes and goods made with tomatoes
Among other leafy greens, spinach
Avocados
Lentils with beans
Foods High in Protein
crimson meat
Chickens
Seafood and fish
Eggs

dairy goods

To develop a customized eating plan that satisfies your nutritional requirements while managing chronic kidney disease (CKD), it's crucial to collaborate with a healthcare professional or a registered dietitian with expertise in kidney disease. To suitably modify dietary recommendations, blood levels and kidney function must be regularly monitored.

FOOD FOR EVERY CKD STAGE

Dietary guidelines for chronic kidney disease (CKD) center on preserving general health, delaying the course of the illness, and treating symptoms. Depending on the stage of CKD, the precise dietary requirements may change, but the following basic recommendations for foods are generally healthy and safe to eat at each stage:

Overarching Recommendations for All CKD
Stages: Low-Sodium Foods

vegetables and fruits that are fresh (in
proper amounts)
Fish, poultry, and fresh meats
popcorn, rice cakes, and nuts are examples
of unsalted snacks (in small amounts)
Foods Low in Phosphorus:

wholesome fruits and veggies
rice milk without added sugar
Non-dairy creamers
Pasta and white bread
Clear and light-colored sodas
Foods Low in Potassium:

Berries, grapes, pineapples, and apples
Lettuce, cabbage, and cauliflower
Pasta, rice, and white bread
cereals made of corn and rice
Moderate Sources of Protein:

Chicken without skin

Trimmed portions of lamb, hog, or cow

eggs, especially the whites

Seafood and fish (in moderation)

Suggestions Specific to Stages

CKD stages 1 and 2

Main Point: Maintain a reasonable protein consumption in a balanced diet, and keep your blood pressure and blood sugar under control.

Foods to Consume: Moderate amounts of fruits and vegetables

Whole grains such as brown rice, barley, and oats

Fish, poultry, and lean meats

dairy products with less fat

Stage 3 CKD

Goals: Start reducing potassium and phosphorus intake, and moderate protein consumption.

Items to Consume: pineapple, berries, apples, and grapes

Radishes, peppers, cauliflower, and cabbage

Bread, spaghetti, and white rice

Egg whites or alternatives to eggs

Trimmed portions of meat and poultry

Stage 4 CKD

Focus: Continue to limit potassium, phosphorus, and protein; regulate fluid intake as necessary.

Consumption: Low-potassium fruits, such as grapes, berries, apples, and cherries

veggies low in potassium, such as cucumbers, green beans, and carrots

Pasta, white rice, and refined grains

Lean meat servings in moderation and egg whites

End-stage renal disease, or CKD, at stage five

Focus: Pay close attention to potassium, phosphorus, and fluid consumption; adjust diet to suit dialysis schedule.

Foods to Eat: Moderate amounts of premium protein (dialysis dependent)

Low-potassium produce and fruits

foods low in phosphorus

Pasta, rice, and white bread

Clear carbonated sodas and low-phosphorus drinks

**Particular Foods to Think About
Fruits:**

Berries (raspberries, blueberries, and raspberries) Apples Plums Pineapples Grapes Vegetables:

cauliflower cabbage
Cucumber Green beans Peppers
Starches and Grains in Zucchini:

Pasta made with white rice
White bread
cereals made of rice
Crackers without salt
Proteins:

Chicken without skin
Lean lamb, hog, or beef chops (in moderation)
Seafood and fish (in moderation)
Egg whites or alternatives to eggs
Alternatives to Dairy:

rice milk without added sugar

Non-dairy creamers

Fluids

Even in the later phases, try to limit your fluid intake while still staying properly hydrated.

Patients with chronic kidney disease (CKD) should collaborate closely with a kidney disease specialist registered dietitian or healthcare practitioner to develop a customized food plan that fits their stage of the disease. For the best possible care, regular monitoring and modifications depending on blood tests and renal function are crucial.

BREAKFAST RECIPES

1. Apple Cinnamon Oatmeal

Ingredients:

- 1/2 cup rolled oats

- 1 cup water
- 1/2 apple, peeled and chopped
- 1/4 teaspoon ground cinnamon
- 1 teaspoon honey or maple syrup (optional)
- 1 tablespoon chopped walnuts (optional, in limited amounts)

Instructions:

1. In a small pot, bring water to a boil.
2. Add rolled oats and chopped apple to the boiling water.
3. Reduce heat to medium and cook for 5-7 minutes, stirring occasionally.
4. Add ground cinnamon and stir well.
5. Remove from heat and let it sit for a minute to thicken.
6. Drizzle with honey or maple syrup if desired.
7. Top with a small amount of chopped walnuts if using.

2. Berry Smoothie

Ingredients:

- 1/2 cup frozen strawberries
- 1/2 cup frozen blueberries
- 1/2 cup rice milk (not enriched) or almond milk (if phosphorus content is low)
- 1/2 cup water
- 1 tablespoon chia seeds (optional, in limited amounts)
- 1 teaspoon honey or agave syrup (optional)

Instructions:

1. Combine all ingredients in a blender.
2. Blend until smooth.
3. Pour into a glass and serve immediately.

3. Veggie Scramble

Ingredients:

- 2 egg whites
- 1/4 cup diced bell peppers

- 1/4 cup diced onions
- 1/4 cup diced zucchini
- 1/4 teaspoon ground black pepper
- 1/2 teaspoon olive oil

Instructions:

1. Heat olive oil in a non-stick skillet over medium heat.
2. Add diced bell peppers, onions, and zucchini to the skillet.
3. Cook vegetables for 3-5 minutes until they are tender.
4. In a small bowl, whisk egg whites with ground black pepper.
5. Pour egg whites into the skillet with the vegetables.
6. Cook, stirring frequently, until the eggs are fully cooked.
7. Serve immediately.

4. Low-Sodium Pancakes

Ingredients:

- 1 cup all-purpose flour

- 1 tablespoon sugar
- 1 teaspoon baking powder
- 1/2 teaspoon baking soda
- 1 cup rice milk (not enriched) or almond milk (if phosphorus content is low)
- 1 egg white
- 1 tablespoon vegetable oil

Instructions:

1. In a large bowl, combine flour, sugar, baking powder, and baking soda.
2. In a separate bowl, whisk together rice milk, egg white, and vegetable oil.
3. Pour the wet ingredients into the dry ingredients and stir until just combined.
4. Heat a non-stick skillet or griddle over medium heat.
5. Pour 1/4 cup of batter onto the skillet for each pancake.
6. Cook until bubbles form on the surface, then flip and cook until golden brown on both sides.

7. Serve with a small amount of honey or maple syrup if desired.

5. Rice Cereal with Berries

Ingredients:

- 1/2 cup rice cereal
- 1 cup water
- 1/4 cup fresh or frozen strawberries, sliced
- 1/4 cup fresh or frozen blueberries
- 1 teaspoon honey or agave syrup (optional)

Instructions:

1. In a small pot, bring water to a boil.
2. Stir in rice cereal and reduce heat to medium-low.
3. Cook, stirring frequently, for 5-7 minutes until thickened.
4. Remove from heat and let it sit for a minute to cool slightly.
5. Top with sliced strawberries and blueberries.

6. Drizzle with honey or agave syrup if desired.
7. Serve warm.

6. Banana Pancakes

Ingredients:

- 1 ripe banana
- 2 egg whites
- 1/4 teaspoon vanilla extract
- 1/4 teaspoon ground cinnamon
- 1/4 teaspoon baking powder
- 1 tablespoon vegetable oil

Instructions:

1. In a bowl, mash the banana until smooth.
2. Add egg whites, vanilla extract, ground cinnamon, and baking powder to the mashed banana and mix until well combined.
3. Heat vegetable oil in a non-stick skillet over medium heat.

4. Pour small amounts of the batter onto the skillet to form pancakes.
5. Cook until bubbles form on the surface, then flip and cook until golden brown on both sides.
6. Serve warm, optionally with a small drizzle of honey or maple syrup.

7. Quinoa Breakfast Bowl

Ingredients:

- 1/2 cup cooked quinoa
- 1/2 apple, peeled and chopped
- 1/4 teaspoon ground cinnamon
- 1 tablespoon chopped walnuts (optional, in limited amounts)
- 1 teaspoon honey or agave syrup (optional)

Instructions:

1. Place cooked quinoa in a bowl.
2. Add chopped apple and ground cinnamon to the quinoa and mix well.
3. Top with chopped walnuts if using.

4. Drizzle with honey or agave syrup if desired.
5. Serve warm.

8. Overnight Chia Pudding

Ingredients:

- 1/4 cup chia seeds
- 1 cup rice milk (not enriched) or almond milk (if phosphorus content is low)
- 1/2 teaspoon vanilla extract
- 1 tablespoon honey or agave syrup (optional)
- 1/4 cup fresh or frozen berries for topping

Instructions:

1. In a bowl or jar, combine chia seeds, milk, vanilla extract, and honey or agave syrup.
2. Stir well to ensure the chia seeds are evenly distributed.
3. Cover and refrigerate overnight.

4. In the morning, stir the chia pudding and top with fresh or frozen berries.
5. Serve chilled.

9. Apple Cinnamon Muffins

Ingredients:

- 1 cup all-purpose flour
- 1/4 cup sugar
- 1/2 teaspoon baking powder
- 1/2 teaspoon baking soda
- 1/4 teaspoon ground cinnamon
- 1/2 cup unsweetened applesauce
- 1/4 cup rice milk (not enriched) or almond milk (if phosphorus content is low)
- 1 egg white
- 1/4 cup finely chopped apples

Instructions:

1. Preheat oven to 350°F (175°C). Line a muffin tin with paper liners.

2. In a large bowl, combine flour, sugar, baking powder, baking soda, and ground cinnamon.
3. In a separate bowl, mix applesauce, milk, and egg white.
4. Pour the wet ingredients into the dry ingredients and stir until just combined.
5. Fold in chopped apples.
6. Divide the batter evenly among the muffin cups.
7. Bake for 20-25 minutes, or until a toothpick inserted into the center comes out clean.
8. Allow to cool before serving.

10. Avocado Toast with Egg Whites

Ingredients:

- 1 slice whole grain bread, toasted
- 1/2 ripe avocado
- 2 egg whites
- 1/4 teaspoon ground black pepper
- 1/4 teaspoon paprika

- 1/2 teaspoon olive oil

Instructions:

1. In a small non-stick skillet, heat olive oil over medium heat.
2. Add egg whites to the skillet and cook until fully set.
3. Mash the avocado and spread it evenly on the toasted bread.
4. Place the cooked egg whites on top of the avocado spread.
5. Sprinkle with ground black pepper and paprika.
6. Serve immediately.

LUNCH RECIPES

1. Grilled Chicken Salad

Ingredients:

- 1 small boneless, skinless chicken breast
- 1 tablespoon olive oil
- 1/4 teaspoon ground black pepper

- 1 teaspoon dried oregano
- 2 cups mixed salad greens (e.g., lettuce, arugula, spinach)
- 1/2 cup cherry tomatoes, halved
- 1/4 cup cucumber, sliced
- 1/4 cup red bell pepper, sliced
- 1 tablespoon lemon juice

Instructions:

1. Preheat a grill or grill pan over medium heat.
2. Brush the chicken breast with olive oil and season with black pepper and dried oregano.
3. Grill the chicken for 5-7 minutes on each side, or until fully cooked.
4. Allow the chicken to rest for a few minutes, then slice into thin strips.
5. In a large bowl, combine salad greens, cherry tomatoes, cucumber, and red bell pepper.
6. Top with grilled chicken slices.
7. Drizzle with lemon juice and serve immediately.

2. Quinoa and Vegetable Stir-Fry

Ingredients:

- 1/2 cup quinoa, rinsed
- 1 cup water
- 1 tablespoon olive oil
- 1/4 cup diced onions
- 1/2 cup diced bell peppers (any color)
- 1/2 cup zucchini, diced
- 1/2 cup broccoli florets
- 1/4 teaspoon ground black pepper
- 1 tablespoon low-sodium soy sauce (optional)

Instructions:

1. In a medium pot, bring water to a boil. Add quinoa, reduce heat to low, cover, and simmer for 15 minutes or until water is absorbed and quinoa is tender.
2. Heat olive oil in a large skillet over medium heat.
3. Add onions and sauté for 2-3 minutes until they begin to soften.

4. Add bell peppers, zucchini, and broccoli to the skillet. Cook for 5-7 minutes, stirring frequently, until vegetables are tender.
5. Add cooked quinoa to the skillet and stir to combine.
6. Season with ground black pepper and low-sodium soy sauce if using.
7. Serve warm.

3. Turkey and Avocado Wrap

Ingredients:

- 1 whole grain tortilla
- 3-4 slices low-sodium deli turkey breast
- 1/4 avocado, thinly sliced
- 1/4 cup shredded lettuce
- 1/4 cup sliced cucumber
- 1 tablespoon hummus (optional)

Instructions:

1. Lay the tortilla flat on a clean surface.

2. Spread hummus evenly over the tortilla if using.
3. Layer turkey slices, avocado, shredded lettuce, and cucumber on the tortilla.
4. Roll the tortilla tightly into a wrap.
5. Slice in half and serve immediately.

4. Lemon Herb Salmon

Ingredients:

- 1 small salmon fillet (about 4 ounces)
- 1 tablespoon olive oil
- 1/4 teaspoon ground black pepper
- 1/2 teaspoon dried dill
- 1 tablespoon lemon juice
- 1 cup steamed green beans or asparagus (for serving)

Instructions:

1. Preheat the oven to 375°F (190°C).
2. Place the salmon fillet on a baking sheet lined with parchment paper.
3. Drizzle with olive oil, and season with ground black pepper and dried dill.

4. Bake for 15-20 minutes, or until the salmon is cooked through and flakes easily with a fork.
5. Remove from the oven and drizzle with lemon juice.
6. Serve with steamed green beans or asparagus.

5. Lentil and Vegetable Soup

Ingredients:

- 1/2 cup dried lentils, rinsed
- 4 cups low-sodium vegetable broth
- 1 tablespoon olive oil
- 1/2 cup diced onions
- 1/2 cup diced carrots
- 1/2 cup diced celery
- 1/2 cup diced tomatoes (fresh or canned, no salt added)
- 1/4 teaspoon ground black pepper
- 1 teaspoon dried thyme

Instructions:

1. Heat olive oil in a large pot over medium heat.
2. Add onions, carrots, and celery. Sauté for 5-7 minutes until vegetables are tender.
3. Add lentils, vegetable broth, diced tomatoes, black pepper, and dried thyme to the pot.
4. Bring to a boil, then reduce heat to low and simmer for 25-30 minutes, or until lentils are tender.
5. Taste and adjust seasoning if necessary.
6. Serve warm.

6. Chickpea Salad

Ingredients:

- 1 cup canned chickpeas, rinsed and drained
- 1/2 cup cherry tomatoes, halved
- 1/4 cup cucumber, diced
- 1/4 cup red bell pepper, diced

- 2 tablespoons red onion, finely chopped
- 1 tablespoon fresh parsley, chopped
- 1 tablespoon olive oil
- 1 tablespoon lemon juice
- 1/4 teaspoon ground black pepper

Instructions:

1. In a large bowl, combine chickpeas, cherry tomatoes, cucumber, red bell pepper, and red onion.
2. In a small bowl, whisk together olive oil, lemon juice, and black pepper.
3. Pour the dressing over the chickpea mixture and toss to combine.
4. Garnish with fresh parsley.
5. Serve chilled or at room temperature.

7. Stuffed Bell Peppers

Ingredients:

- 2 medium bell peppers (any color)
- 1/2 cup cooked quinoa

- 1/4 cup cooked lean ground turkey or beef
- 1/4 cup diced tomatoes (fresh or canned, no salt added)
- 1/4 cup diced zucchini
- 1/4 teaspoon ground black pepper
- 1/2 teaspoon dried basil
- 1 tablespoon olive oil

Instructions:

1. Preheat the oven to 375°F (190°C).
2. Cut the tops off the bell peppers and remove the seeds and membranes.
3. In a large bowl, combine cooked quinoa, ground turkey or beef, diced tomatoes, zucchini, black pepper, and dried basil.
4. Stuff the bell peppers with the quinoa mixture.
5. Place the stuffed peppers in a baking dish and drizzle with olive oil.
6. Cover with foil and bake for 25-30 minutes, or until the peppers are tender.

7. Serve warm.

8. Chicken and Vegetable Skewers

Ingredients:

- 1 boneless, skinless chicken breast, cut into bite-sized pieces
- 1/2 red bell pepper, cut into chunks
- 1/2 yellow bell pepper, cut into chunks
- 1/2 zucchini, cut into slices
- 1/4 red onion, cut into chunks
- 2 tablespoons olive oil
- 1 tablespoon lemon juice
- 1 teaspoon dried oregano
- 1/4 teaspoon ground black pepper

Instructions:

1. Preheat the grill to medium-high heat.
2. In a large bowl, combine olive oil, lemon juice, dried oregano, and black pepper.
3. Add chicken pieces to the bowl and toss to coat.

4. Thread the chicken, bell peppers, zucchini, and red onion onto skewers.

5. Grill the skewers for 10-15 minutes, turning occasionally, until the chicken is cooked through and the vegetables are tender.

6. Serve immediately.

9. Baked Cod with Herbs

Ingredients:

- 1 cod fillet (about 4 ounces)
- 1 tablespoon olive oil
- 1/4 teaspoon ground black pepper
- 1/2 teaspoon dried thyme
- 1 tablespoon lemon juice
- 1/4 cup steamed green beans (for serving)

Instructions:

1. Preheat the oven to 375°F (190°C).

2. Place the cod fillet on a baking sheet lined with parchment paper.

3. Drizzle with olive oil and season with black pepper and dried thyme.
4. Bake for 15-20 minutes, or until the cod is cooked through and flakes easily with a fork.
5. Remove from the oven and drizzle with lemon juice.
6. Serve with steamed green beans.

10. Veggie Pasta Salad

Ingredients:

- 1 cup cooked whole grain pasta
- 1/2 cup cherry tomatoes, halved
- 1/4 cup cucumber, diced
- 1/4 cup red bell pepper, diced
- 1/4 cup black olives, sliced (optional)
- 1 tablespoon olive oil
- 1 tablespoon red wine vinegar
- 1/4 teaspoon ground black pepper
- 1/2 teaspoon dried oregano

Instructions:

1. In a large bowl, combine cooked pasta, cherry tomatoes, cucumber, red bell pepper, and black olives if using.
2. In a small bowl, whisk together olive oil, red wine vinegar, black pepper, and dried oregano.
3. Pour the dressing over the pasta salad and toss to combine.
4. Serve chilled or at room temperature.

DINNER RECIPES

1. Baked Lemon Herb Chicken

Ingredients:

- 2 boneless, skinless chicken breasts
- 2 tablespoons olive oil
- 1 tablespoon lemon juice
- 1 teaspoon dried rosemary
- 1 teaspoon dried thyme
- 1/4 teaspoon ground black pepper
- 2 cloves garlic, minced
- 1 cup steamed broccoli (for serving)

Instructions:

1. Preheat the oven to 375°F (190°C).
2. In a small bowl, mix olive oil, lemon juice, dried rosemary, dried thyme, black pepper, and minced garlic.
3. Place the chicken breasts in a baking dish and pour the herb mixture over them, ensuring they are well-coated.
4. Bake for 25-30 minutes, or until the chicken is cooked through and juices run clear.
5. Serve with steamed broccoli.

2. Vegetable Stir-Fry with Tofu

Ingredients:

- 1 block firm tofu, drained and cubed
- 1 tablespoon olive oil
- 1/2 cup sliced bell peppers (any color)
- 1/2 cup broccoli florets
- 1/2 cup snap peas
- 1/4 cup sliced carrots
- 2 tablespoons low-sodium soy sauce
- 1/4 teaspoon ground black pepper
- 1 teaspoon grated fresh ginger

- 1 cup cooked white rice (for serving)

Instructions:

1. Heat olive oil in a large skillet over medium-high heat.
2. Add cubed tofu and cook until golden brown on all sides, about 5-7 minutes. Remove tofu from the skillet and set aside.
3. In the same skillet, add bell peppers, broccoli, snap peas, and carrots. Stir-fry for 5-7 minutes until vegetables are tender-crisp.
4. Return tofu to the skillet. Add low-sodium soy sauce, black pepper, and grated ginger. Stir well to combine.
5. Serve over cooked white rice.

3. Garlic Shrimp and Asparagus

Ingredients:

- 1 pound large shrimp, peeled and deveined

- 1 bunch asparagus, trimmed and cut into 2-inch pieces
- 2 tablespoons olive oil
- 3 cloves garlic, minced
- 1/4 teaspoon ground black pepper
- 1 tablespoon lemon juice
- 1/4 cup chopped fresh parsley (optional)

Instructions:

1. Heat olive oil in a large skillet over medium-high heat.
2. Add minced garlic and sauté for 1-2 minutes until fragrant.
3. Add shrimp and asparagus to the skillet. Cook, stirring frequently, until the shrimp are pink and opaque, and the asparagus is tender, about 5-7 minutes.
4. Season with black pepper and lemon juice. Stir well to combine.
5. Garnish with chopped fresh parsley if desired.
6. Serve immediately.

4. Turkey Meatballs with Zucchini Noodles

Ingredients:

- 1 pound ground turkey
- 1/4 cup breadcrumbs (use low-sodium or homemade)
- 1 egg white
- 1/4 cup grated Parmesan cheese (optional, in limited amounts)
- 2 cloves garlic, minced
- 1 teaspoon dried oregano
- 1/4 teaspoon ground black pepper
- 2 tablespoons olive oil
- 4 zucchinis, spiralized into noodles
- 1 cup low-sodium marinara sauce (optional)

Instructions:

1. In a large bowl, combine ground turkey, breadcrumbs, egg white, Parmesan cheese (if using), minced

garlic, dried oregano, and black pepper. Mix well.

2. Form the mixture into small meatballs.

3. Heat olive oil in a large skillet over medium heat. Add the meatballs and cook until browned on all sides and cooked through, about 10-12 minutes. Remove meatballs from the skillet and set aside.

4. In the same skillet, add spiralized zucchini noodles and cook for 3-4 minutes until slightly tender.

5. If using marinara sauce, heat it in a separate saucepan over medium heat.

6. Serve meatballs over zucchini noodles, with marinara sauce if desired.

5. Baked Cod with Roasted Vegetables

Ingredients:

- 2 cod fillets (about 4 ounces each)
- 2 tablespoons olive oil
- 1 tablespoon lemon juice

- 1 teaspoon dried thyme
- 1/4 teaspoon ground black pepper
- 1 cup cherry tomatoes, halved
- 1 cup zucchini, sliced
- 1 cup bell peppers, sliced
- 1/2 red onion, sliced

Instructions:

1. Preheat the oven to 400°F (200°C).
2. In a small bowl, mix olive oil, lemon juice, dried thyme, and black pepper.
3. Place cod fillets on a baking sheet lined with parchment paper. Brush the cod fillets with the olive oil mixture.
4. On a separate baking sheet,

place cherry tomatoes, zucchini, bell peppers, and red onion. Drizzle with a little olive oil and season with black pepper. 5. Place both the cod and the vegetables in the oven. 6. Bake the vegetables for 20-25 minutes, stirring halfway through. 7. Bake the cod for 15-20 minutes, or until the fish flakes easily with a fork. 8. Serve the baked cod with the roasted vegetables.

6. Stuffed Bell Peppers with Quinoa and Veggies

Ingredients:

- 2 large bell peppers (any color)
- 1/2 cup cooked quinoa
- 1/4 cup chopped tomatoes (fresh or canned, no salt added)
- 1/4 cup finely chopped zucchini
- 1/4 cup finely chopped mushrooms
- 1/4 cup chopped onions
- 1 tablespoon olive oil
- 1/4 teaspoon ground black pepper
- 1 teaspoon dried basil
- 1/4 cup shredded low-fat mozzarella cheese (optional, in limited amounts)

Instructions:

1. Preheat the oven to 375°F (190°C).
2. Cut the tops off the bell peppers and remove the seeds and membranes.

3. In a skillet, heat olive oil over medium heat. Add onions, zucchini, mushrooms, and tomatoes. Cook for 5-7 minutes until vegetables are tender.
4. Stir in cooked quinoa, black pepper, and dried basil. Mix well.
5. Stuff the bell peppers with the quinoa mixture.
6. Place the stuffed peppers in a baking dish. Top with shredded cheese if using.
7. Cover with foil and bake for 25-30 minutes, or until the peppers are tender.
8. Serve warm.

7. Lemon Herb Grilled Salmon

Ingredients:

- 2 salmon fillets (about 4 ounces each)
- 2 tablespoons olive oil
- 1 tablespoon lemon juice
- 1 teaspoon dried dill

- 1/4 teaspoon ground black pepper
- 1 cup steamed green beans (for serving)

Instructions:

1. Preheat the grill to medium-high heat.
2. In a small bowl, mix olive oil, lemon juice, dried dill, and black pepper.
3. Brush the salmon fillets with the olive oil mixture.
4. Grill the salmon for 4-5 minutes on each side, or until the fish flakes easily with a fork.
5. Serve with steamed green beans.

8. Turkey and Veggie Lettuce Wraps

Ingredients:

- 1/2 pound ground turkey
- 1 tablespoon olive oil
- 1/2 cup diced bell peppers
- 1/2 cup diced zucchini
- 1/4 cup diced onions

- 1 teaspoon low-sodium soy sauce (optional)
- 1/4 teaspoon ground black pepper
- 1 teaspoon grated fresh ginger
- 8 large lettuce leaves (e.g., romaine or butter lettuce)

Instructions:

1. Heat olive oil in a large skillet over medium heat.
2. Add diced onions and cook for 2-3 minutes until softened.
3. Add ground turkey to the skillet and cook until browned, about 5-7 minutes.
4. Stir in bell peppers, zucchini, black pepper, and grated ginger. Cook for an additional 5-7 minutes until vegetables are tender.
5. Add low-sodium soy sauce if using, and stir well.
6. Spoon the turkey and vegetable mixture into large lettuce leaves.
7. Serve immediately.

9. Baked Tilapia with Herbs and Lemon

Ingredients:

- 2 tilapia fillets (about 4 ounces each)
- 2 tablespoons olive oil
- 1 tablespoon lemon juice
- 1/4 teaspoon ground black pepper
- 1 teaspoon dried thyme
- 1 cup steamed asparagus (for serving)

Instructions:

1. Preheat the oven to 375°F (190°C).
2. Place the tilapia fillets on a baking sheet lined with parchment paper.
3. In a small bowl, mix olive oil, lemon juice, black pepper, and dried thyme.
4. Brush the tilapia fillets with the olive oil mixture.
5. Bake for 15-20 minutes, or until the fish flakes easily with a fork.
6. Serve with steamed asparagus.

10. Beef and Vegetable Kebabs

Ingredients:

- 1/2 pound lean beef, cut into bite-sized pieces
- 1/2 cup cherry tomatoes
- 1/2 cup zucchini, sliced
- 1/2 cup bell peppers, cut into chunks
- 1/4 cup red onions, cut into chunks
- 2 tablespoons olive oil
- 1 tablespoon balsamic vinegar
- 1 teaspoon dried oregano
- 1/4 teaspoon ground black pepper

Instructions:

1. Preheat the grill to medium-high heat.
2. In a bowl, mix olive oil, balsamic vinegar, dried oregano, and black pepper.
3. Thread the beef, cherry tomatoes, zucchini, bell peppers, and red onions onto skewers.
4. Brush the kebabs with the olive oil mixture.

5. Grill the kebabs for 10-15 minutes, turning occasionally, until the beef is cooked to your liking and the vegetables are tender.
6. Serve immediately.

1. Apple Slices with Almond Butter

Ingredients:

- 1 medium apple, sliced
- 2 tablespoons almond butter (ensure it's low in sodium and no added sugar)

Instructions:

1. Wash and slice the apple into thin wedges.
2. Spread almond butter evenly on each apple slice.
3. Serve immediately as a quick and healthy snack.

2. Cucumber and Hummus Bites

Ingredients:

- 1 large cucumber, sliced into rounds
- 1/2 cup hummus (low sodium)
- 1 tablespoon fresh dill, chopped (optional, for garnish)

Instructions:

1. Wash and slice the cucumber into 1/4-inch thick rounds.
2. Place a small dollop of hummus on each cucumber slice.
3. Garnish with fresh dill if desired.
4. Serve immediately.

3. Berry Yogurt Parfait

Ingredients:

- 1/2 cup plain Greek yogurt (low phosphorus and low potassium if possible)
- 1/4 cup fresh blueberries
- 1/4 cup fresh strawberries, sliced

- 1 tablespoon honey or agave syrup (optional)

Instructions:

1. In a small bowl or glass, layer half of the yogurt.
2. Add half of the blueberries and strawberries on top of the yogurt layer.
3. Repeat with the remaining yogurt and berries.
4. Drizzle with honey or agave syrup if desired.
5. Serve immediately or refrigerate until ready to eat.

4. Rice Cakes with Avocado Spread

Ingredients:

- 2 plain rice cakes (low sodium)
- 1/2 ripe avocado
- 1/4 teaspoon ground black pepper
- 1/4 teaspoon lemon juice

Instructions:

1. In a small bowl, mash the avocado with a fork.
2. Add ground black pepper and lemon juice to the mashed avocado and mix well.
3. Spread the avocado mixture evenly over the rice cakes.
4. Serve immediately.

5. Carrot and Celery Sticks with Greek Yogurt Dip

Ingredients:

- 1 cup carrot sticks
- 1 cup celery sticks
- 1/2 cup plain Greek yogurt (low phosphorus and low potassium if possible)
- 1 teaspoon lemon juice
- 1/2 teaspoon dried dill
- 1/4 teaspoon ground black pepper

Instructions:

1. In a small bowl, mix the Greek yogurt,
   lemon juice, dried dill, and ground
   black pepper to make the dip.
2. Arrange the carrot and celery sticks on
   a plate.
3. Serve the veggies with the Greek
   yogurt dip on the side.

6. Cottage Cheese and Pineapple Cups

Ingredients:

- 1/2 cup low-fat cottage cheese
- 1/4 cup diced pineapple (fresh or
  canned in juice, drained)
- 1 tablespoon chopped fresh mint
  (optional)

Instructions:

1. In a small bowl, mix together cottage
   cheese and diced pineapple.
2. Spoon the mixture into small serving
   cups.
3. Garnish with chopped fresh mint if
   desired.

4. Serve immediately.

7. Roasted Chickpeas

Ingredients:

- 1 can (15 ounces) chickpeas (garbanzo beans), drained and rinsed
- 1 tablespoon olive oil
- 1/2 teaspoon ground cumin
- 1/2 teaspoon paprika
- 1/4 teaspoon garlic powder
- 1/4 teaspoon salt (optional)

Instructions:

1. Preheat the oven to 400°F (200°C) and line a baking sheet with parchment paper.
2. Pat the chickpeas dry with a paper towel and place them on the prepared baking sheet.
3. Drizzle with olive oil and sprinkle with ground cumin, paprika, garlic powder, and salt if using. Toss to coat evenly.

4. Spread the chickpeas out in a single layer.
5. Bake for 20-30 minutes, stirring occasionally, until golden and crispy.
6. Allow to cool before serving.

8. Rice Cake with Tuna Salad

Ingredients:

- 1 rice cake (low sodium)
- 1/4 cup canned tuna, drained
- 1 tablespoon plain Greek yogurt (low phosphorus and low potassium if possible)
- 1 tablespoon chopped cucumber
- 1 tablespoon chopped red bell pepper
- 1/2 teaspoon lemon juice
- 1/4 teaspoon dried dill
- Salt and pepper to taste (optional)

Instructions:

1. In a small bowl, mix together canned tuna, Greek yogurt, chopped cucumber, chopped red bell pepper,

lemon juice, dried dill, salt, and pepper if using.
2. Spread the tuna salad mixture onto the rice cake.
3. Serve immediately.

9. Veggie Chips

Ingredients:

- 1 large sweet potato, thinly sliced
- 1 large beet, thinly sliced
- 1 tablespoon olive oil
- 1/4 teaspoon garlic powder
- 1/4 teaspoon onion powder
- Salt to taste (optional)

Instructions:

1. Preheat the oven to 375°F (190°C) and line a baking sheet with parchment paper.
2. In a bowl, toss sweet potato and beet slices with olive oil, garlic powder, onion powder, and salt if using.

3. Arrange the slices in a single layer on the prepared baking sheet.
4. Bake for 20-25 minutes, flipping halfway through, until the chips are crispy.
5. Allow to cool before serving.

10. Greek Yogurt Bark

Ingredients:

- 1 cup plain Greek yogurt (low phosphorus and low potassium if possible)
- 1 tablespoon honey or maple syrup (optional)
- 1/4 cup mixed berries (e.g., blueberries, strawberries, raspberries)

Instructions:

1. Line a baking sheet with parchment paper.
2. In a bowl, mix together Greek yogurt and honey or maple syrup if using.

3. Spread the Greek yogurt mixture evenly onto the prepared baking sheet.
4. Sprinkle mixed berries over the top.
5. Freeze for 2-3 hours, or until firm.
6. Break into pieces before serving.

1. Baked Apples with Cinnamon

Ingredients:

- 2 apples
- 1 tablespoon unsalted butter, melted
- 1/2 teaspoon ground cinnamon
- 1 tablespoon chopped walnuts (optional, in limited amounts)

Instructions:

1. Preheat the oven to 375°F (190°C).
2. Core the apples and remove the seeds, leaving the bottom intact.
3. Place the apples in a baking dish.
4. In a small bowl, mix melted butter and ground cinnamon.

5. Brush the cinnamon butter mixture over the apples, ensuring they are evenly coated.
6. Bake for 20-25 minutes, or until the apples are tender.
7. Remove from the oven and sprinkle chopped walnuts over the top if using.
8. Serve warm.

2. Berry Parfait

Ingredients:

- 1/2 cup low-fat Greek yogurt (low phosphorus and low potassium if possible)
- 1/4 cup mixed berries (e.g., blueberries, strawberries, raspberries)
- 1 tablespoon crushed low-sodium graham crackers or granola

Instructions:

1. In a glass or bowl, layer half of the Greek yogurt.

2. Add half of the mixed berries on top of the yogurt layer.
3. Repeat with the remaining yogurt and berries.
4. Sprinkle crushed graham crackers or granola over the top.
5. Serve immediately.

3. Frozen Banana Bites

Ingredients:

- 1 ripe banana
- 2 tablespoons unsalted almond butter or peanut butter (check for low sodium)
- 2 tablespoons dark chocolate chips (optional, in limited amounts)

Instructions:

1. Peel the banana and cut it into thin slices.
2. Spread almond butter or peanut butter on half of the banana slices.

3. Top with the remaining banana slices to form sandwiches.
4. Place the banana sandwiches on a baking sheet lined with parchment paper.
5. Melt dark chocolate chips in the microwave or on the stovetop using a double boiler.
6. Drizzle melted chocolate over the banana sandwiches.
7. Freeze for 1-2 hours, or until firm.
8. Serve frozen.

4. Chia Seed Pudding

Ingredients:

- 2 tablespoons chia seeds
- 1/2 cup unsweetened almond milk or rice milk (low phosphorus and low potassium if possible)
- 1/4 teaspoon vanilla extract
- 1 tablespoon honey or maple syrup (optional)

- Fresh fruit for topping (e.g., sliced strawberries, blueberries)

Instructions:

1. In a bowl or jar, mix chia seeds, almond milk or rice milk, vanilla extract, and honey or maple syrup if using.
2. Stir well to combine.
3. Cover and refrigerate overnight, or for at least 2-3 hours, until the mixture thickens.
4. Stir the chia seed pudding and top with fresh fruit before serving.

5. Grilled Pineapple with Cinnamon

Ingredients:

- 1 fresh pineapple, peeled and cored
- 1 tablespoon honey (optional)
- 1/2 teaspoon ground cinnamon

Instructions:

1. Preheat a grill or grill pan over medium-high heat.
2. Cut the pineapple into rings or wedges.
3. Brush each pineapple slice with honey if using.
4. Sprinkle ground cinnamon over the pineapple slices.
5. Grill the pineapple slices for 2-3 minutes on each side, or until grill marks appear.
6. Serve warm.

6. Peach and Cottage Cheese Bowl

Ingredients:

- 1 ripe peach, sliced
- 1/2 cup low-fat cottage cheese
- 1 tablespoon chopped almonds (optional, in limited amounts)
- 1 teaspoon honey or agave syrup (optional)

Instructions:

1. Arrange peach slices in a bowl.
2. Top with low-fat cottage cheese.
3. Sprinkle chopped almonds over the top if using.
4. Drizzle with honey or agave syrup if desired.
5. Serve immediately.

7. Frozen Yogurt Bark with Fruit

Ingredients:

- 1 cup plain Greek yogurt (low phosphorus and low potassium if possible)
- 1 tablespoon honey or maple syrup (optional)
- 1/4 cup mixed berries (e.g., blueberries, raspberries)
- 1/4 cup chopped mango or pineapple

Instructions:

1. Line a baking sheet with parchment paper.

2. In a bowl, mix together Greek yogurt and honey or maple syrup if using.
3. Spread the Greek yogurt mixture evenly onto the prepared baking sheet.
4. Sprinkle mixed berries and chopped mango or pineapple over the top.
5. Freeze for 2-3 hours, or until firm.
6. Break into pieces before serving.

8. Lemon Sorbet

Ingredients:

- 2 cups water
- 1/2 cup fresh lemon juice
- 1/4 cup honey or agave syrup
- 1 tablespoon lemon zest
- Fresh mint leaves for garnish (optional)

Instructions:

1. In a saucepan, combine water, lemon juice, honey or agave syrup, and lemon zest.

2. Heat over medium heat, stirring until the sweetener is dissolved.
3. Remove from heat and let cool to room temperature.
4. Pour the mixture into a shallow dish and freeze for about 4-6 hours, stirring every hour with a fork to break up ice crystals.
5. Once frozen, scrape the mixture with a fork to create a sorbet-like texture.
6. Serve in bowls or glasses, garnished with fresh mint leaves if desired.

9. Chocolate Avocado Mousse

Ingredients:

- 1 ripe avocado
- 2 tablespoons unsweetened cocoa powder
- 2 tablespoons honey or maple syrup
- 1/2 teaspoon vanilla extract
- Pinch of salt (optional)
- Fresh berries for topping (e.g., raspberries, strawberries)

Instructions:

1. Scoop the flesh of the avocado into a blender or food processor.
2. Add cocoa powder, honey or maple syrup, vanilla extract, and salt if using.
3. Blend until smooth and creamy.
4. Transfer the mousse to serving bowls or glasses.
5. Refrigerate for at least 30 minutes before serving.
6. Top with fresh berries before serving.

10. Coconut Rice Pudding

Ingredients:

- 1/2 cup uncooked white rice
- 2 cups unsweetened coconut milk
- 1/4 cup honey or maple syrup
- 1 teaspoon vanilla extract
- 1/4 teaspoon ground cinnamon
- Unsweetened shredded coconut for garnish (optional)

Instructions:

1. In a saucepan, combine uncooked white rice, coconut milk, honey or maple syrup, vanilla extract, and ground cinnamon.
2. Bring to a boil over medium heat, then reduce heat to low and simmer for 20-25 minutes, stirring occasionally, until the rice is cooked and the mixture has thickened.
3. Remove from heat and let cool slightly.
4. Transfer the rice pudding to serving bowls.
5. Sprinkle with unsweetened shredded coconut for garnish if desired.
6. Serve warm or chilled.

BEVERAGES RECIPES

1. Cucumber Mint Cooler

Ingredients:

- 1 cucumber, peeled and sliced
- 1/4 cup fresh mint leaves

- 4 cups water
- 1 tablespoon honey or agave syrup (optional)
- Ice cubes

Instructions:

1. In a blender, combine cucumber slices, mint leaves, water, and honey or agave syrup if using.
2. Blend until smooth.
3. Strain the mixture through a fine mesh sieve to remove any pulp.
4. Chill in the refrigerator for at least 1 hour.
5. Serve over ice cubes.

2. Ginger Lemon Iced Tea

Ingredients:

- 4 cups water
- 2-inch piece fresh ginger, peeled and thinly sliced
- 2 green tea bags
- 1 lemon, thinly sliced

- 1 tablespoon honey or agave syrup (optional)
- Ice cubes

Instructions:

1. In a saucepan, bring water to a boil.
2. Add sliced ginger and green tea bags to the boiling water.
3. Remove from heat and let steep for 5-7 minutes.
4. Strain the tea to remove ginger slices and tea bags.
5. Allow the tea to cool to room temperature.
6. Stir in lemon slices and honey or agave syrup if using.
7. Chill in the refrigerator for at least 1 hour.
8. Serve over ice cubes.

3. Watermelon Lime Fresca

Ingredients:

- 2 cups cubed seedless watermelon

- Juice of 2 limes
- 2 cups water
- 1 tablespoon honey or agave syrup (optional)
- Ice cubes
- Fresh mint leaves for garnish (optional)

Instructions:

1. In a blender, combine cubed watermelon, lime juice, water, and honey or agave syrup if using.
2. Blend until smooth.
3. Strain the mixture through a fine mesh sieve to remove any pulp.
4. Chill in the refrigerator for at least 1 hour.
5. Serve over ice cubes and garnish with fresh mint leaves if desired.

4. Berry Blast Smoothie

Ingredients:

- 1/2 cup mixed berries (e.g., strawberries, blueberries, raspberries)
- 1/2 cup low-fat plain Greek yogurt (low phosphorus and low potassium if possible)
- 1/2 cup unsweetened almond milk or rice milk (low phosphorus and low potassium if possible)
- 1 tablespoon honey or agave syrup (optional)
- Ice cubes

Instructions:

1. In a blender, combine mixed berries, Greek yogurt, almond milk or rice milk, and honey or agave syrup if using.
2. Blend until smooth.
3. Add ice cubes and blend again until desired consistency is reached.
4. Serve immediately.

5. Herbal Iced Tea

Ingredients:

- 4 cups water
- 2 herbal tea bags (e.g., chamomile, peppermint, or rooibos)
- 1 tablespoon honey or agave syrup (optional)
- Ice cubes
- Lemon slices for garnish (optional)

Instructions:

1. In a saucepan, bring water to a boil.
2. Remove from heat and add herbal tea bags.
3. Let steep for 5-7 minutes.
4. Remove tea bags and allow the tea to cool to room temperature.
5. Stir in honey or agave syrup if using.
6. Chill in the refrigerator for at least 1 hour.
7. Serve over ice cubes with lemon slices for garnish if desired.

1. Vegetable and Quinoa Soup

Ingredients:

- 1 tablespoon olive oil
- 1 onion, chopped
- 2 cloves garlic, minced
- 2 carrots, diced
- 2 celery stalks, diced
- 1 zucchini, diced
- 1/2 cup quinoa, rinsed
- 6 cups low-sodium vegetable broth
- 1 teaspoon dried thyme
- 1/2 teaspoon dried oregano
- Salt and pepper to taste
- Fresh parsley for garnish (optional)

Instructions:

1. Heat olive oil in a large pot over medium heat.
2. Add chopped onion and minced garlic. Sauté until fragrant, about 2 minutes.

3. Add diced carrots, celery, and zucchini. Cook for another 5 minutes.
4. Stir in rinsed quinoa, vegetable broth, dried thyme, and dried oregano.
5. Bring the soup to a boil, then reduce heat and simmer for 15-20 minutes, or until quinoa and vegetables are tender.
6. Season with salt and pepper to taste.
7. Garnish with fresh parsley if desired before serving.

2. Chicken and Rice Soup

Ingredients:

- 1 tablespoon olive oil
- 1 onion, chopped
- 2 cloves garlic, minced
- 2 carrots, diced
- 2 celery stalks, diced
- 1 cup cooked chicken breast, shredded
- 1/2 cup white rice
- 6 cups low-sodium chicken broth
- 1 teaspoon dried thyme

- Salt and pepper to taste
- Fresh parsley for garnish (optional)

Instructions:

1. Heat olive oil in a large pot over medium heat.
2. Add chopped onion and minced garlic. Sauté until fragrant, about 2 minutes.
3. Add diced carrots and celery. Cook for another 5 minutes.
4. Stir in shredded chicken breast, white rice, chicken broth, and dried thyme.
5. Bring the soup to a boil, then reduce heat and simmer for 15-20 minutes, or until rice and vegetables are tender.
6. Season with salt and pepper to taste.
7. Garnish with fresh parsley if desired before serving.

3. Lentil and Spinach Soup

Ingredients:

- 1 tablespoon olive oil
- 1 onion, chopped

- 2 cloves garlic, minced
- 1 carrot, diced
- 1 celery stalk, diced
- 1 cup dry green or brown lentils, rinsed
- 6 cups low-sodium vegetable broth
- 2 cups fresh spinach leaves
- 1 teaspoon ground cumin
- 1/2 teaspoon ground coriander
- Salt and pepper to taste
- Lemon wedges for serving (optional)

Instructions:

1. Heat olive oil in a large pot over medium heat.
2. Add chopped onion and minced garlic. Sauté until fragrant, about 2 minutes.
3. Add diced carrot and celery. Cook for another 5 minutes.
4. Stir in rinsed lentils, vegetable broth, ground cumin, and ground coriander.
5. Bring the soup to a boil, then reduce heat and simmer for 20-25 minutes, or until lentils are tender.

6. Stir in fresh spinach leaves and cook until wilted, about 2-3 minutes.
7. Season with salt and pepper to taste.
8. Serve with lemon wedges for squeezing over the soup if desired.

4. Tomato Basil Soup

Ingredients:

- 1 tablespoon olive oil
- 1 onion, chopped
- 2 cloves garlic, minced
- 2 cans (14 ounces each) diced tomatoes (no salt added)
- 4 cups low-sodium vegetable broth
- 1/4 cup chopped fresh basil leaves
- Salt and pepper to taste
- Freshly grated Parmesan cheese for garnish (optional)

Instructions:

1. Heat olive oil in a large pot over medium heat.

2. Add chopped onion and minced garlic.
    Sauté until fragrant, about 2 minutes.
3. Add diced tomatoes (with their juices)
    and vegetable broth.
4. Bring the soup to a boil, then reduce
    heat and simmer for 15-20 minutes.
5. Stir in chopped fresh basil leaves.
6. Using an immersion blender or
    regular blender, blend the soup until
    smooth.
7. Season with salt and pepper to taste.
8. Serve hot, garnished with freshly
    grated Parmesan cheese if desired.

5. Potato Leek Soup

Ingredients:

- 2 tablespoons unsalted butter
- 2 leeks, white and light green parts only, sliced
- 2 cloves garlic, minced
- 3 large potatoes, peeled and diced
- 4 cups low-sodium vegetable broth
- 1 cup low-fat milk

- Salt and pepper to taste
- Chopped chives for garnish (optional)

Instructions:

1. In a large pot, melt butter over medium heat.
2. Add sliced leeks and minced garlic. Sauté until softened, about 5 minutes.
3. Add diced potatoes and vegetable broth to the pot.
4. Bring the soup to a boil, then reduce heat and simmer for 20-25 minutes, or until potatoes are tender.
5. Using an immersion blender or regular blender, blend the soup until smooth.
6. Stir in low-fat milk and heat through.
7. Season with salt and pepper to taste.
8. Serve hot, garnished with chopped chives if desired.

BONUS

1. Garlic Roasted Green Beans

Ingredients:

- 1 pound fresh green beans, trimmed
- 2 tablespoons olive oil
- 3 cloves garlic, minced
- Salt and pepper to taste

Instructions:

1. Preheat the oven to 400°F (200°C).
2. In a large bowl, toss green beans with olive oil, minced garlic, salt, and pepper until evenly coated.
3. Spread the green beans in a single layer on a baking sheet.
4. Roast in the preheated oven for 15-20 minutes, or until tender and slightly browned, stirring halfway through.
5. Serve hot.

2. Lemon Garlic Roasted Broccoli

Ingredients:

- 1 pound broccoli florets
- 2 tablespoons olive oil
- 2 cloves garlic, minced
- Zest of 1 lemon
- Salt and pepper to taste

Instructions:

1. Preheat the oven to 400°F (200°C).
2. In a large bowl, toss broccoli florets with olive oil, minced garlic, lemon zest, salt, and pepper until evenly coated.
3. Spread the broccoli in a single layer on a baking sheet.
4. Roast in the preheated oven for 15-20 minutes, or until tender and lightly browned, stirring halfway through.
5. Serve hot.

3. Balsamic Glazed Carrots

Ingredients:

- 1 pound carrots, peeled and sliced into sticks
- 2 tablespoons olive oil
- 2 tablespoons balsamic vinegar
- 1 tablespoon honey or maple syrup
- Salt and pepper to taste

Instructions:

1. Preheat the oven to 400°F (200°C).
2. In a large bowl, toss carrot sticks with olive oil, balsamic vinegar, honey or maple syrup, salt, and pepper until evenly coated.
3. Spread the carrots in a single layer on a baking sheet.
4. Roast in the preheated oven for 20-25 minutes, or until tender and caramelized, stirring halfway through.
5. Serve hot.

4. Stir-Fried Sesame Garlic Bok Choy

Ingredients:

- 1 pound baby bok choy, halved or quartered
- 2 tablespoons olive oil
- 2 cloves garlic, minced
- 1 tablespoon low-sodium soy sauce
- 1 tablespoon toasted sesame oil
- Sesame seeds for garnish (optional)

Instructions:

1. Heat olive oil in a large skillet or wok over medium-high heat.
2. Add minced garlic and sauté for 1 minute, or until fragrant.
3. Add bok choy to the skillet and stir-fry for 4-5 minutes, or until tender-crisp.
4. Drizzle low-sodium soy sauce and toasted sesame oil over the bok choy, tossing to coat evenly.
5. Cook for another 1-2 minutes.
6. Remove from heat and sprinkle with sesame seeds if desired before serving.

5. Oven-Roasted Brussels Sprouts

Ingredients:

- 1 pound Brussels sprouts, trimmed and halved
- 2 tablespoons olive oil
- 2 cloves garlic, minced
- Salt and pepper to taste

Instructions:

1. Preheat the oven to 400°F (200°C).
2. In a large bowl, toss Brussels sprouts with olive oil, minced garlic, salt, and pepper until evenly coated.
3. Spread the Brussels sprouts in a single layer on a baking sheet.
4. Roast in the preheated oven for 20-25 minutes, or until tender and caramelized, stirring halfway through.
5. Serve hot.

APPETIZER AND HEALTHY RECIPE
BONUS

1. Stuffed Bell Peppers

Ingredients:

- 4 bell peppers (any color)
- 1 cup cooked quinoa
- 1 can (15 ounces) low-sodium black beans, drained and rinsed
- 1 cup diced tomatoes
- 1/2 cup diced onion
- 1/2 cup corn kernels (fresh, frozen, or canned)
- 1/2 teaspoon ground cumin
- 1/2 teaspoon chili powder
- Salt and pepper to taste
- 1/2 cup shredded low-fat cheese (optional)

Instructions:

1. Preheat the oven to 375°F (190°C) and line a baking dish with parchment paper.
2. Cut the tops off the bell peppers and remove the seeds and membranes.
3. In a large bowl, mix together cooked quinoa, black beans, diced tomatoes,

diced onion, corn kernels, ground cumin, chili powder, salt, and pepper.

4. Stuff the bell peppers with the quinoa mixture and place them in the prepared baking dish.
5. If using, sprinkle shredded cheese on top of each stuffed pepper.
6. Cover the baking dish with aluminum foil and bake for 25-30 minutes, or until the peppers are tender.
7. Remove the foil and bake for an additional 5-10 minutes, or until the cheese is melted and bubbly.
8. Serve hot.

2. Cucumber Roll-Ups

Ingredients:

- 1 large cucumber
- 1/2 cup low-fat cream cheese or Greek yogurt cream cheese
- 1/4 cup diced bell pepper (any color)
- 1/4 cup shredded carrots
- 1/4 cup sliced black olives

- Salt and pepper to taste
- Fresh herbs for garnish (optional)

Instructions:

1. Slice the cucumber lengthwise into thin strips using a mandoline slicer or vegetable peeler.
2. In a small bowl, mix together low-fat cream cheese, diced bell pepper, shredded carrots, sliced black olives, salt, and pepper.
3. Spread a thin layer of the cream cheese mixture onto each cucumber strip.
4. Roll up the cucumber strips and secure with toothpicks if necessary.
5. Garnish with fresh herbs if desired before serving.

3. Hummus Stuffed Mini Peppers

Ingredients:

- 10 mini bell peppers (any color)
- 1/2 cup hummus (low sodium)

- 1/4 cup diced cucumber
- 1/4 cup diced tomatoes
- 1/4 cup chopped fresh parsley
- Salt and pepper to taste

Instructions:

1. Cut the tops off the mini bell peppers and remove the seeds and membranes.
2. Fill each pepper with a spoonful of hummus.
3. Top with diced cucumber, diced tomatoes, and chopped fresh parsley.
4. Season with salt and pepper to taste.
5. Serve chilled or at room temperature.

4. Spinach and Feta Stuffed Mushrooms

Ingredients:

- 10 large button mushrooms, stems removed and reserved
- 1 tablespoon olive oil
- 2 cloves garlic, minced

- 2 cups fresh spinach leaves, chopped
- 1/4 cup crumbled feta cheese
- Salt and pepper to taste

Instructions:

1. Preheat the oven to 375°F (190°C) and line a baking sheet with parchment paper.
2. Finely chop the reserved mushroom stems.
3. Heat olive oil in a skillet over medium heat.
4. Add minced garlic and chopped mushroom stems to the skillet. Sauté until softened, about 3-4 minutes.
5. Add chopped spinach to the skillet and cook until wilted, about 2-3 minutes.
6. Remove from heat and stir in crumbled feta cheese. Season with salt and pepper to taste.
7. Spoon the spinach and feta mixture into the mushroom caps.
8. Place the stuffed mushrooms on the prepared baking sheet.

9. Bake for 15-20 minutes, or until the mushrooms are tender and the filling is golden brown.

10. Serve warm.

5. Avocado and Tomato Salsa

Ingredients:

- 2 ripe avocados, diced
- 1 cup diced tomatoes
- 1/4 cup diced red onion
- 1/4 cup chopped fresh cilantro
- 1 jalapeño, seeded and minced (optional)
- Juice of 1 lime
- Salt and pepper to taste
- Baked tortilla chips for serving

Instructions:

1. In a large bowl, gently combine diced avocados, diced tomatoes, diced red onion, chopped fresh cilantro, and minced jalapeño if using.

2. Squeeze lime juice over the avocado mixture and toss gently to coat.
3. Season with salt and pepper to taste.
4. Serve with baked tortilla chips for dipping.

Day 1:

Breakfast:

- Scrambled Egg Whites with Spinach and Tomatoes
- Whole Grain Toast
- Sliced Cantaloupe

Lunch:

- Quinoa Salad with Chickpeas, Cucumbers, and Bell Peppers
- Low-fat Greek Yogurt

Dinner:

- Baked Salmon with Lemon and Dill
- Steamed Asparagus

- Brown Rice

Day 2:

Breakfast:

- Overnight Oats with Chia Seeds, Berries, and Almond Milk

Lunch:

- Lentil Soup
- Mixed Green Salad with Balsamic Vinaigrette

Dinner:

- Grilled Chicken Breast
- Roasted Brussels Sprouts
- Quinoa Pilaf

Day 3:

Breakfast:

- Whole Grain Pancakes with Fresh Berries

- Unsweetened Applesauce

Lunch:

- Turkey and Avocado Wrap with Whole Wheat Tortilla
- Carrot Sticks with Hummus

Dinner:

- Vegetable Stir-Fry with Tofu
- Brown Rice

Day 4:

Breakfast:

- Greek Yogurt Parfait with Granola and Sliced Banana

Lunch:

- Spinach and Feta Stuffed Mushrooms
- Mixed Berry Salad with Lemon Poppyseed Dressing

Dinner:

- Baked Cod with Herbed Quinoa
- Steamed Green Beans

Day 5:

Breakfast:

- Breakfast Burrito with Scrambled Eggs, Black Beans, and Salsa

Lunch:

- Chicken Caesar Salad with Homemade Dressing (Low Sodium)

Dinner:

- Turkey Meatballs with Marinara Sauce
- Whole Wheat Pasta
- Steamed Broccoli

Day 6:

Breakfast:

- Smoothie Bowl with Spinach, Banana, Greek Yogurt, and Almond Butter

Lunch:

- Tuna Salad Lettuce Wraps
- Sliced Watermelon

Dinner:

- Vegetable and Bean Chili
- Cornbread (Low Sodium)

Day 7:

Breakfast:

- Oatmeal with Sliced Almonds and Diced Apples

Lunch:

- Quinoa and Black Bean Stuffed Bell Peppers

Dinner:

- Grilled Steak (Lean Cuts)
- Roasted Sweet Potatoes
- Steamed Asparagus

Day 8:

Breakfast:

- Whole Grain Toast with Mashed Avocado
- Poached Egg
- Sliced Strawberries

Lunch:

- Turkey and Vegetable Soup
- Whole Grain Crackers

Dinner:

- Grilled Shrimp Skewers
- Quinoa Salad with Cherry Tomatoes and Cucumber
- Steamed Green Beans

Day 9:

Breakfast:

- Greek Yogurt with Honey and Almonds

- Whole Grain Granola

Lunch:

- Chicken and Vegetable Stir-Fry with Brown Rice

Dinner:

- Baked Halibut with Garlic and Herbs
- Roasted Cauliflower
- Wild Rice Pilaf

Day 10:

Breakfast:

- Spinach and Feta Crustless Quiche

Lunch:

- Lentil and Vegetable Salad with Lemon-Tahini Dressing

Dinner:

- Turkey Chili with Kidney Beans
- Cornbread Muffin (Low Sodium)

Day 11:

Breakfast:

- Smoothie with Spinach, Banana, Berries, and Almond Milk

Lunch:

- Tuna and White Bean Salad
- Sliced Peaches

Dinner:

- Baked Chicken Breast with Rosemary and Lemon
- Roasted Root Vegetables
- Couscous

Day 12:

Breakfast:

- Whole Grain Waffles with Fresh Fruit Compote (No Added Sugar)

Lunch:

- Egg Salad Lettuce Wraps
- Carrot and Celery Sticks with Hummus

Dinner:

- Vegetable and Tofu Curry
- Brown Rice

Day 13:

Breakfast:

- Cottage Cheese Pancakes with Blueberry Compote (No Added Sugar)

Lunch:

- Spinach and Chickpea Salad with Balsamic Vinaigrette

Dinner:

- Grilled Salmon with Dill Sauce
- Steamed Asparagus
- Quinoa Pilaf

Day 14:

Breakfast:

- Breakfast Burrito with Scrambled Eggs, Black Beans, Avocado, and Salsa

Lunch:

- Caprese Salad with Fresh Mozzarella, Tomato, and Basil

Dinner:

- Beef and Vegetable Kabobs
- Grilled Zucchini
- Whole Wheat Couscous

Day 15:

Breakfast:

- Spinach and Mushroom Omelette
- Whole Grain Toast
- Sliced Orange

Lunch:

- Quinoa and Black Bean Salad with Lime Vinaigrette

Dinner:

- Grilled Chicken Breast
- Roasted Brussels Sprouts
- Brown Rice

Day 16:

Breakfast:

- Greek Yogurt Parfait with Granola and Sliced Banana

Lunch:

- Lentil Soup
- Mixed Green Salad with Balsamic Vinaigrette

Dinner:

- Baked Cod with Herbed Quinoa
- Steamed Green Beans

Day 17:

Breakfast:

- Smoothie Bowl with Spinach, Banana, Greek Yogurt, and Almond Butter

Lunch:

- Chicken Caesar Salad with Homemade Dressing (Low Sodium)

Dinner:

- Turkey Meatballs with Marinara Sauce
- Whole Wheat Pasta
- Steamed Broccoli

Day 18:

Breakfast:

- Overnight Oats with Chia Seeds, Berries, and Almond Milk

Lunch:

- Spinach and Feta Stuffed Mushrooms

- Mixed Berry Salad with Lemon Poppyseed Dressing

Dinner:

- Vegetable and Bean Chili
- Cornbread (Low Sodium)

Day 19:

Breakfast:

- Whole Grain Pancakes with Fresh Berries
- Unsweetened Applesauce

Lunch:

- Turkey and Avocado Wrap with Whole Wheat Tortilla
- Carrot Sticks with Hummus

Dinner:

- Baked Salmon with Lemon and Dill
- Steamed Asparagus
- Brown Rice

Day 20:

Breakfast:

- Oatmeal with Sliced Almonds and Diced Apples

Lunch:

- Quinoa and Black Bean Stuffed Bell Peppers

Dinner:

- Grilled Steak (Lean Cuts)
- Roasted Sweet Potatoes
- Steamed Asparagus

Day 21:

Breakfast:

- Whole Grain Toast with Mashed Avocado
- Poached Egg
- Sliced Strawberries

Lunch:

- Turkey and Vegetable Soup
- Whole Grain Crackers

Dinner:

- Grilled Shrimp Skewers
- Quinoa Salad with Cherry Tomatoes and Cucumber
- Steamed Green Beans

Day 22:

Breakfast:

- Spinach and Feta Crustless Quiche

Lunch:

- Lentil and Vegetable Salad with Lemon-Tahini Dressing

Dinner:

- Baked Halibut with Garlic and Herbs
- Roasted Cauliflower

- Wild Rice Pilaf

Day 23:

Breakfast:

- Greek Yogurt with Honey and Almonds
- Whole Grain Granola

Lunch:

- Chicken and Vegetable Stir-Fry with Brown Rice

Dinner:

- Turkey Chili with Kidney Beans
- Cornbread Muffin (Low Sodium)

Day 24:

Breakfast:

- Smoothie with Spinach, Banana, Berries, and Almond Milk

Lunch:

- Tuna and White Bean Salad
- Sliced Peaches

Dinner:

- Baked Chicken Breast with Rosemary and Lemon
- Roasted Root Vegetables
- Couscous

Day 25:

Breakfast:

- Whole Grain Waffles with Fresh Fruit Compote (No Added Sugar)

Lunch:

- Egg Salad Lettuce Wraps
- Carrot and Celery Sticks with Hummus

Dinner:

- Vegetable and Tofu Curry
- Brown Rice

Day 26:

Breakfast:

- Cottage Cheese Pancakes with Blueberry Compote (No Added Sugar)

Lunch:

- Spinach and Chickpea Salad with Balsamic Vinaigrette

Dinner:

- Grilled Salmon with Dill Sauce
- Steamed Asparagus
- Quinoa Pilaf

Day 27:

Breakfast:

- Breakfast Burrito with Scrambled Eggs, Black Beans, Avocado, and Salsa

Lunch:

- Caprese Salad with Fresh Mozzarella, Tomato, and Basil

Dinner:

- Beef and Vegetable Kabobs
- Grilled Zucchini
- Whole Wheat Couscous

Day 28:

Breakfast:

- Scrambled Egg Whites with Spinach and Tomatoes
- Whole Grain Toast
- Sliced Cantaloupe

Lunch:

- Quinoa Salad with Chickpeas, Cucumbers, and Bell Peppers
- Low-fat Greek Yogurt

Dinner:

- Baked Salmon with Lemon and Dill

- Steamed Asparagus
- Brown Rice

Day 29:

Breakfast:

- Overnight Oats with Chia Seeds, Berries, and Almond Milk

Lunch:

- Lentil Soup
- Mixed Green Salad with Balsamic Vinaigrette

Dinner:

- Grilled Chicken Breast
- Roasted Brussels Sprouts
- Brown Rice

Day 30:

Breakfast:

- Greek Yogurt Parfait with Granola and Sliced Banana

Lunch:

- Chicken Caesar Salad with Homemade Dressing (Low Sodium)

Dinner:

- Turkey Meatballs with Marinara Sauce
- Whole Wheat Pasta
- Steamed Broccoli

CONCLUSION

In conclusion, a CKD diet cookbook tailored for all stages of chronic kidney disease offers a comprehensive range of recipes designed to support kidney health while providing delicious and satisfying meals. By focusing on nutrient balance, portion control, and the incorporation of kidney-friendly ingredients, such a cookbook empowers individuals with CKD to manage their condition through mindful eating choices. From breakfast to dinner, and even snacks and desserts, these recipes offer variety and flavor while adhering to dietary restrictions associated with CKD. With the guidance of a healthcare provider or dietitian, individuals can utilize this cookbook as a valuable resource in promoting kidney health and overall well-being throughout their CKD journey.

THE END